Lil Girl ~ Grown Woman

Lil Girl ~ Grown Woman

By

Levonda Carter-Versailles

Please find my other books

Remember The Times

On The Road with Peaches

Email: <u>mybooksin2016@yahoo.com</u>
Website:
http://whitehouzeproduction.wix.com/levondacarter

Dedication

I would like to dedicate this short story book to those young girls that may be on the way to losing themselves.

I also would like to dedicate this story to the women that have children; please be a great role model and teach your children. Set an example. For those that have HIV, Life isn't OVER!
Seek Help!

ACKNOWLEDGEMENTS

I would like to thank God for Blessing me and my family. I thank Him for keeping me safe through all the hard times in my life.

I thank my husband, Mr. Versailles, for believing in me and sticking in there with me during all of the crazy things that I've done. Love you Husband.

I thank all of my friends, family and readers who support me on my journey as a new writer.

I thank, Authoress Loretta Morris White, for assisting me with the Publishing of my books.

FORWARD

Young women now a days are growing up real fast. They are out of control. They're doing this and that. There's nothing no one can do about it either, it seems. It's just sad and this is why I came up with this story.

Things I see other woman do these days make me think and realize how great of a woman I am. I see women with four to five baby daddy's. I say to myself; when will they ever learn and when will they ever realize that these men are not here for them?

They care about get what they only care for and leave you struggling by yourself.

I was raised in a family where my mother had 3 kids by 3 different men and trust me, as a child, life was hard. So really ladies, think about what your child will go through. I told myself I would never let this happen because what you do as a child or as you get older, it will influence your children. So try and think about what they will go through and try to change what our kids are doing in this century.

In this chapter you will learn about Tracy, is a young girl trying hard to be like her mother and the other older teenagers. She is about 12 years old. She has friends that are older than she is. Lisa and Kiki, are in their early teens; Fourteen years of age and every one else is a lot older than they are.

You will learn so much about the mother, Kathy. She is heavily on drugs. She also works for her son, Jason, as a Prostitute. Jason is a Pimp and runs the house. Jason's younger sister is in that stage of getting into a lot of trouble. So as you see, this is how it goes.

Chapter 1

Today it's hot and sunny out. The kids are outside playing; momma's out on the porch playing cards and having some beer, listing to some old school music with her friends. Mom is a single woman that's on drugs bad and all I wanted to do is be like the grown women I see in my hood. They have all kinds of men and all kinds of money flowing through the house.

Tracy is thinking this in her head. She doesn't know that her mom is on drugs, but she knows her mom smokes and sit at home all day.

Her moms' friends are in and out of the house with a different man. Tracy wants to pick up the habit as well.

Tracy asks her mom if she could go play outside with her friend. Her mom tells her, "Go on child don't you see grown folks out here talking and stuff." Her mom yells at her and she runs off.

Tracy ran off over to see her friends, Lisa and Kiki, they both have kids. Well each of them have one child and would you think that she is headed in the wrong direction.

Well while Tracy sitting on this little lounge chair at Kiki house, some older boy named CJ comes up and holler at her. She has been having a crush on CJ for quite some time now. Her friends happen to run into him one day and told him that Tracy has a crush on him. Tracy didn't know that yet so she is happy about it not knowing that they using her to get money for them, see how friends do you wrong?

Poor Tracy, she is about to have a rude wakening soon and she hardly even know CJ.

CJ is now up in her face sweet talking her and they are hugging and kissing already on the first day. She tells him she in love with him and he's saying the same thing but really he knows what time it is.

Well out of nowhere, Kiki comes running out the house and is fighting some other girl in the street. Tracy run out to have Kiki back, making sure that no one jumps in the fight.

CJ is telling Tracy not to jump in someone else fight. Tracy says no, that's her friend and to let her go.

Lisa runs out now and come to find out, they were fighting over a boy. The boy was sleeping with another girl after he had been with Kiki.

Kiki saw the girl out side and wanted to fight her because of her baby daddy. Kiki and Lisa's mom came out to break up the fight.

They told them that they need to be looking for jobs and to stop wondering what these men were out here doing with the next woman. "They are all dogs", Kiki and Lisa mom said.

So Tracy says, "Awww man, y'all got to go inside now it's getting dark and y'all need to start walking me home."

So now she's mad because Kiki and Lisa mom wont let them back out the door. So the boy

CJ says, "I'll walk you home. Aren't you just around the corner?" He asks.

Tracy says, "Yes what, you gonna walk me home? But you can't tell my mom and my brother that we talking."

CJ says, "Talking! Girl we dating." She smiles and they began to walk.

Her momma is calling her, telling her to get her fast ass home right now.

She yells back into the phone. "Mom I'm right around the corner! I'm coming."

Tracy and CJ meets her mom and they introduce themselves. "I'm Miss Kathy. Boy who are you, bringing my daughter home? Where are her friends at that supposed to bring her home?"

CJ says, "Well they were in a fight and their mom asked me to bring her home, so here she is Miss Kathy your loving daughter."

Miss Kathy says, "oh ok thank you for that." Miss Kathy ask him if he wanted to stay for a little while. He says yes he sure will.

Her mom said she had to run off with her son Jason, and that he was waiting for her to come. She didn't want to keep Jason waiting, that's what she tells Tracy.

She tells Tracy not to let anyone else in the house because she's going out for the night. She said she will send Jason by the house to check up on her in an hour.

Tracy tells her mom goodbye and to go ahead. "I'm good." So her mom leaves.

Now do you see what is wrong with this picture? An older boy alone in the house with your soft hearted daughter that's crazy.

But people will learn, unless its them. As an adult we're not supposed to do that. I don't care how bad you wanna go out. Ain't no way in the world! Oh well lesson learned.

So CJ and Tracy is sitting on the couch touching and kissing and rubbing all over each other. They're making out and Tracy begin to take off her clothes, she asks CJ if her body look good to him.

He says, "Yes, for your age you have some nice pretty breast and a nice round ass.

She smiles and let him feel her up. He tells her to turn around and pull her pink panties off. She does and say wait, do you have a condom (at 12 what you know about a condom?)

So as he tells her, "Oh don't worry I'm not trying to get you pregnant, I just want to teach you some grown woman things." CJ says to Tracy. (shame, just sad)

And of course she ready for what he wants to show her. He slowly puts it in her Vagina. She tells him it hurts her and he says of course its going to hurt for a moment first because its your first time. She's telling him to stop and take it easy he yells at her and say, "Whore you know you want it!"

He gets off her and begin to get a little ruff with her. She starts to cry at that moment, wanting him to stop but he doesn't. He turns her over and begin to have anal sex with her. She yells for help but no one hears her cry for help. He finishes what he's doing and pull up his paints and put on his shirt.

He tells Tracy, "Now that's how you handle being a grown woman."

She says, "No its not! you hurt me. I don't like what you done to me.

"Oh so what you thought, this was a game out here?" He yells at her. "And if you tell anyone I promise you that I'll kill you."

"No you won't!" she responds.

He slaps her in the face. "You better watch your mouth. Now you work for me. My little whore."

Now she's afraid and say, "No I'm not!

He says, "Oh what you think your friends do for me and why you think their mom so cool with me? It's because I help them make a living where they live. They are my whores too and they hooked me up with you." He adds.

Tracy starts to cry and tells him that he lying.

He say, "Ok ask them." She says, no she don't want to deal with nobody and for him to get out of her house.

He tells her fine. But before he leaves, he says remember what I said.

She says, "whatever!"

He tells her to go clean herself up. "You're bleeding all over yourself." And she shut her door.

As CJ is leaving out the house, her big brother, Jason comes up and question him.

"Yo, man what the fuck you doing coming out my house?" Jason shows his gun and it scares CJ.

"Yo man, ya moms told me to chill with lil momma till you came to check on her. She told me to look out for you, homie." CJ says to Jason.

Jason says, "Oh ok dawg, no sweat you cool. Thanks for looking out." CJ leaves the house.

Tracy looks at her brother and say to him, "Yo, why u didn't kick his ass?" She mumbles while crying.

He asks, "What Tracy, home boy said y'all was cool and all. Why what happened?" He yells at Tracy.

She tells him that she was raped by CJ, that's what happened.

Jason ran out to try and catch him but CJ had already gone not to be found, not yet. Jason ran back in the house and said that he is going to kill him for hurting his sister.

She says, "No because he will kill me and I'm scared to get our family involved in my mess."

Only Tracy knew what to do in order for her family to be safe.

The only thing she knew and saw what CJ had told her what the deal was is what she had to do. She told Jason and he told her that she's going to school and gonna make something of herself, that she was not going to be anyone's whore.

She said, "No I can't go back, he'll look for me at the school."

So now Tracy is stuck with having to be a slut of the town where she's from. Jason is pissed off and says to Tracy they will figure out a plan and that they can't tell nobody what she is doing.

Jason says he'll look out for her. Jason tells Tracy to get cleaned up and they're going out, so she can see what's going on out in these streets.

(Hey like they say don't keep wishing for things you really don't want to happen).

Tracy has always wished to be an adult but now looks like she moved too fast. Poor Tracy.

Well its now midnight and Tracy and her brother hit the streets and ran into their mom. Tracy asked, "Mom what you doing out here?

She said, "getting fast money!" She never wanted her daughter to know what she was doing, but Tracy had a clue when she saw men in and out of their home, and other people partying every night.

It was causing her not to be able to focus on her school work. She was too busy trying to see what was going on. Well guess what, Tracy got a taste of her medicine.

Her mom asks, "What are you doing out and where is that boy at that was with you?"

Tracy respond, "It's a long story mom."

Her mom tells her, "Well go back home and go to bed.

She said, "I can't mom." She begins to cry.

Her mom asks, "What's wrong, what happened?"

Jason says, "She got raped into a gang that her two friends were in. She didn't know until he raped her in the ass."

Her mother was very upset and out of control. She yelled, "Oh no, we're going to the hospital to get you checked out."

The brother says, "That's not all, he told her that she also got to work for him out here to get money." Jason said that he was going to look out for her out here like he does his mother.

Her mother said, "Well you in a gang now and nothing I can do about it." She also told Tracy to watch her friends because they already had kids young. She should have known that if they didn't have a job, and they just were out at night.

Well Tracy got some rude awakening. She was that blind not to see that she can get out if she wanted, but she didn't so she got what she wanted.

Of course she got raped more and used more and lost things, she was homeless at times, she'd get tired of dealing with her friends and would run away. It got to the point that she was depressed and almost killed herself like her mom did.

So when it got that far some one found her laid out on the road and took her to the hospital and stood by her till she was better.

She was on drugs really bad and almost overdosed. Then she was treated back in a crazy home (mental hospital), and realized this life wasn't for her. So she stayed in the crazy home for quite some time till the doctor thought she was ok to be out on her own.

But before all that, she got into a low income housing program to help her to get on her feet. She also found out that she was HIV positive, and it was from CJ. It had started in her anal area. That's where CJ mostly had sex with her and raping her. The Doctor wanted to press charges on CJ because he was having sex with a minor and infecting her along with other underage girls and women, with HIV.

But no one would come forward to the court to come clean about him. Only one, Tracy first friend. She was raped as well and ended up with HIV. She didn't tell any of her partners because she didn't know until she got pregnant.

So thank God that her baby was not infected. They got the drugs in the baby just in time so it bypassed the baby.

Now CJ is put away and Tracy is starting a new life.

So now let's see, what going on in this next chapter.

Chapter 2: Tracy new life trying to keep clean.

Well Tracy gets clean for a while. She was put into a home under Government help due to the fact of her finding out she has H. I. V. from CJ nasty ass. Her friend went and filed charges on him when she knew she had it as well, but she could not get no one else to help her. So Tracy came up and told her, well CJ is now put away for spreading HIV.

The girls came up with a plan and started a club for those that had been raped and was on drugs and had HIV.

In order to capture the ones that aren't telling that they have HIV, they'd go out and do speeches on HIV and every thing and to let a partner know they have it.

Yes, some were scared for their lives but a Law was passed where; if you don't tell, you'd do time in prison. Some would and some didn't. Some fought for their lives, some were killed but the girls did what it took to try and let it slow down.

So the government helped them out with a place and car to get around to get the club going. They were doing good,

Tracy's other friend was killed in a shooting. Tracy other friend boyfriend at the time was taking care of the baby also that one doesn't have HIV, but the mother do. The boyfriend does as well so he was also coming aboard the club to help out, even though he had a job. He just wanted to support them because they all had HIV.

So time goes on a while, Tracy began writing a book to become an author. Her friend died of HIV, she had given up on her life. She didn't want to live in pain any longer.

Tracy moved on and supported the group no matter what happen because she didn't want this to keep happening to others.

Well as time goes on, she also gave up because she realized that she could not stop it. People just don't care, so she did write a book about her story; it's titled, "If time can kill."

Well time went by and Kathy went to Lakeside Mental Health, after 2 years of not seeing her brother or mother and letting them know what had been happening with her.

She went by to see her mother Kathy. She did not really want to go see her but she had a change of heart about her mother and said she need to help her and go get checked. Well the mother didn't have HIV, but she did. She wasn't being careful at all when it came to her body, but she went to Lakeside and told her mother what had happen since she was a lil girl.

Kathy, the mother was listening and she seemed more stable to listen than she ever was before. It felt good to Tracy to be able to sit and talk after 3 long years of being off drugs, so they talked and talked and had lunch.

The doctor said that they won't let her mother out till she at least has done 5 years clean. Then they'll put her in a living environment with a roommate and be included in a work program. They wanted to make sure that she would be in a stable environment. She will be in the program for a year, if she fails a test she will do 5-6 years in prison.

So as time went on, her and the mother are doing ok. But there's one thing that she has to face as well; the fact that the guy CJ may get out, if they can't get someone else to come up and speak again. Someone else has complained about CJ doing this. They wanna put him in the chair, on death row now, so there is still more to come in this case.

Tracy is scared that he will get out and come for her. Tracy said she has to move again, where no one knows her nor can find her if she has to go through this again.

She said yes, to the officer that she will do everything to keep him out the streets and from doing this to anyone again if it kills her.

Tracy visits her mom again, her mom is in a Drug free-living program and is doing good but the brother has 2 more years in prison. He'll be out soon as well. He is on a work program too so he can get a job but I guess you will hear about that part in the next chapter.

So as you see, this family is on a serious rollercoaster. But eventually, in it all, they seem to try and pull together as a family.

Well time has come for Tracy to see the Judge and say what he had done to her, in order to help the young lady, keep him behind bars.

The trial went on for months before they came to a decision. But Tracy wasn't worried she had a plan. If he did come out, she said she wasn't running anymore from nobody ever again in her life.

She did face him in court and they won the case. Now CJ will be on death row because of how many women he had infected. Most of them didn't know until they were seen by a doctor.

Time had passed and people will watch CJ die in the chair and give his last words. His last words were, "All woman deserve to die if they're a whore!" And he smiled with an evil smile and laughed as he died.

So there was no more CJ he's gone for good. Poor nasty CJ.

Well Tracy has asked God for forgiveness if she had given anyone HIV. Tracy has to live with this all her life. It is up to Tracy to make sure she's safe when doing things but she is good. She has no kids and no man in her life at the moment. She is helping her mother keep clean for their living program they're in also.

Now she decides that she has to go and start seeing her brother Jason, who is still locked up as well. He's still trying to get out and to do better.

But like I say, we will get into Jason's story later on in the book. So back to Tracy.

She is now living with HIV, her friend is doing good as well but like I said; the other was killed in a shooting well she killed herself, basically.

Tracy goes out with her mother to eat, she is looking nice and as they sit down to eat people stare at them, "like wow is that them!" as if they got a makeover. But, how long is this going to last in everyone's head?

The whole town know how Tracy and her mom are and if not, they have heard it from everything being on the news.

Well they know that Tracy is HIV positive. Well most of them do, but Tracy is enjoying time with her mother.

A nice looking young man, around Tracy age, walks up and starts looking her up and down. He was like, "damn ma, look at you!"

She slaps him because on the streets she knew what that meant and she told him to respect her. She's a woman now. Come to find out that was what he was trying to tell Tracy. She apologized. It's just the fact, "I know how men are."

This young man said, "Well all men aren't the same."

Tracy smiles and think, for the first time in her life he was the first person that had said something nice to her.

He joined them for dinner. Tracy admitted to him that she was HIV. He says so that's a good thing then, because he found out he had HIV too.

As you see, there is somebody for everybody in this world.

People need to be a lot more careful because you never know what you can get. Most people may not tell the truth unless they're in trouble, or if they get caught.

So as you see Tracy is getting her life back on track so far, yes so far. The mother is on a probation period, where she can't be out too late because of the program that's helping her get her housing back. She has three more months before they give her own place back again.

As time goes on, Tracy is now dating this man and people are wondering or don't understand how she has a man in her life but not knowing that both of them have HIV.

People always want to know about the next person so much. Tracy and her new guy would go out and enjoy themselves. Sometimes they'd beat up on Tracy because people knew her. But they didn't know about her friend. Her friend would help out and one day, he all-of-a sudden yelled out to the entire public that he has HIV as well. He asked people to stop bugging them please and people froze up, and looked at them as he yelled.

He was fed up and said, "Any one got a problem, fight me. We are still people that just got messed up." He said "You can't get it if we hug or touch you or cough, the only way is through sex and needles so please stop it!"

It won't change how people feel and are scared of it so if you scared of it then maybe and hopefully people will realize that they need to strap up twice and be careful this time in the world.

Well as time moves on, Tracy is still with her boyfriend she had shared some stories to him letting him know her past. He didn't care because he had a rough time as well and so now they have moved in with each other.

Looks like things are going good so far. Oh but don't get ya hope up just yet. There is more to come that he's going to want her to do. Trust that they are going to have it out bad, but that's coming up soon as well.

Tracy still can't find work, the boyfriend is getting feed up with lack of work so things are getting hard. She got off the program she was on because she was working but that wasn't enough for extra things in the house. When she got with her boyfriend, she moved with him not realizing that she messed herself up again.

The boyfriend told her that she might need to be a stripper again but this time no sex with men. She told him, no and she didn't want to be reminded of her past ever again so he slapped her for talking back and he said she had no choice.

Chapter 3

Tracy and her boyfriend started working the clubs and she goes back to stripping. Her brother Jason is released.

Let's see how this goes, more drama to come, poor Tracy, and all her problems. It's going down and Tracy's back to the money. Ain't this a bitch! Oh well.

So Tracy and her new man are in a hole somehow. Tracy got to find out why they stopped her housing. Well I think she really knows why; it's supposed to be for single women with HIV. She figured that it would be ok.

They saw that there was more income when living with a man. So now she has to get a job and it was hard for her to get one so fast. Her man said without him working that many hours she'd have to go back dancing for a while.

Tracy said, "No!" And cried her eyes out to her man.

He said, "Honey it's just for a while till we get on our feet."

She gave in and said ok and that's how she got back into dancing. So fucked up! She gave in and there you have it.

So she went to the club where she used to dance at and no one knew she had HIV at this point in life, she didn't care anymore anyway.

Tracy ran into an old friend that she used to walk the streets with. Not her old friend, that had died long ago. Her friend said, "Girl I thought you died."

She says, "No I just left for a while to get myself back on track."

"Well it must didn't go well."

"It did for a while but things were hard for me at my old job and bills were falling behind. So here I am back to square one."

So her friend says, "Well welcome back to this hell-hole club, quick money it is. But we got to do what we got to do."

So she out working the club getting back high on drugs so that she can feel better doing her job.

It's hard doing this, she thinks. She shed a tear. Tracy says, Fuck it! I got to pull up my grown woman panties and hit this floor. So out she walks with a see-through dress, white bra and panties on and clear light up pumps, a gold lace front wig and her face made-up. So she'd hit the dance floor and shake her ass off. She made over a thousand dollars. Well, guess she knew what the men liked.

Tracy worked all night and sometimes a double if she had to. She started to really feel herself and she didn't feel like a little girl anymore she was now a grown woman.

Well I guess you know, Tracy now pays all the bills and she don't walk the streets no more she just dances every night.

It's to the point her boyfriend beats on her for sex and she don't have time for it but he beats her till she passes out and she gives in again after a while. Tracy is feed up and is ready to go in flip mode. Tracy, at this point goes to shooting classes to get a gun in her name. She runs into her brother and she asks him for a gun. He sees her and looks at her face and asked why she let those men beat on and rape her.

She told him, that she knows he isn't talking. She says, "You used to beat on your tricks."

And he replied, "But Tracy you not a trick you my lil sister."

"Well it's the same thing as if you were doing it too." She says he's no better than the rest if he does it too.

He says, "Ok Tracy you got a point there but its work."

Tracy says, "Bullshit that's a street job! I know because I was a street walker remember."

He laughs at her and say, "Yeah sis, but you grown now, and I'm not gonna beat my woman no more. But he can't help the hustle that's out here right now in this world he says. So he asks Tracy what she need a gun for, she says the same reason that you need one.

So he takes her to shooting class so she can get her own permit. He says, "that boyfriend of yours must be doing this, if you not messing with no one he says if he is, fry his ass if he does it again."

She says, that's why she need it. So she gets hers on and she goes on with her day. Back to the club and then her boyfriend shows up to check on her. Y'all know what that means, yes more drama to come.

Well that night, she didn't want to fight with him any more, so she gave him what she had so far to pay their bills. Tracy felt like she was back at where she tried to leave from the start, but she got sucked back in and not only that, she was helping her brother out as well.

To tell you the truth I don't feel bad for some one that keep thinking that there's nothing that they can't do but get quick, fast money.

I don't understand how you go back to square one and knowing you have HIV or you've caught something from it. If you don't like the fact of what you doing well damn it, change your life style stop making up excuses for yourself.

It's a lot more to life than fast money the nasty way life can be. So it's great if you just have faith and give it a chance. Yes, you'll have a few bumps in the road, but that mean you've passed God's test that's all. Any way just was a lil talk back to the story.

So Tracy said, fuck it she'd pop a pill called Molly, so she'd be high and have her a drink and get really drunk. She didn't want to feel nothing because of what she was out doing.

She began to work the streets more with her brother at night and at day she was at the club until 1:00am. Then the streets with her brother, like wow how can you do that?

She met a girl named Candy. Her old friends were gone and when she met Candy it was like her and her friend all over again. Candy was a mix woman that also had HIV so they didn't care about anything anymore.

The boyfriend had both of them and she didn't mind. Her brother was protecting them as well. All the boy friend did was just watch and join some man, he is as you can see; his sorry ass was on chill mode and had other women while she was out as well.

Ummmm, SMH, poor Tracy done went crazy and began to be just like her mother but worse.

Like I say it's up to you to get out of this mess on your own after a while.

Tracy got tired of having a man so she caught her boyfriend and kicked him out and told him he didn't have to do it behind her back she would have let the women join in. She was already into other women from when she stripped at the club.

So he left but she was still with Candy so I guess she felt better now lol. Her and Candy went off to work at the club. The club was called Chocolate City nothing but mostly black went there, a few whites work there but it was more of a shake your booty club and boom room. And it was a big body guard.

Well at least for quite some time she was doing her and was in love with Candy. They were doing good. It was to the point where the brother ended up back in jail and they had a bigger place. Big time men even were using them in shows and still no one cares about that these women had HIV.

The world has gone mad and you have to be careful now adays.

So one day she ends up in the hospital because she was attacked really bad. Candy was pulling her weight to keep the bills up as always.

Tracy was in a coma for about 2 months in God hands she woke up and couldn't remember anything.

Tracy and Candy was good with each other and now that they came up with that new law that Gays can be married well as you see that they went and got married.

Tracy got better and gave up stripping and came up with her own church group since there wasn't a church yet that let Gays in so as y'all know.

Tracy got better, yes she was still HIV her and Candy were also. Candy was still a stripper but instead of her out she did things in the club and no, Candy didn't believe in church like Tracy did.

One-day Tracy woke up and began to write a book about her life all over again. But this one was like her second one of herself and how she had learned about the fast life of coming into the life of the streets.

Well this is Tracy new life, oh by the way her Brother gets out of jail and get shot at but not sure if he is crippled or in a wheel chair. I believe he starts slowing down after the bad shooting and everything.

Tracy began to look out for her brother and yes, Candy old self, now is still a stripper and Tracy is a self-published Author that works at a store.

Well as time go on you live life and you learn people make mistakes in life. Nobody is perfect so don't judge people you never know what can happen. Just keep focused and keep moving on tending to yourself.

In this chapter you will see that Tracy is taking care of her brother and the brother will die. She lost her mother over HIV and drugs, her mother was doing good at first. But it's the streets of life this chapter is also about Tracy and Candy getting into a big fight and what you think it was about? Well I'll leave that for you'll to keep reading on.

Chapter 4 The Life of the Streets

Tracy tell about her life, it's just a little bit about her brother that she can say. He didn't want to get his life together and he ends up getting HIV as well. He doesn't care who he ends up sleeping with. He also ends up getting shot. All because of Candy.

Candy gets home one night, she tells Tracy that her bother got shot and killed.

Tracy ask "Why, what happened?"

Candy's screaming and yelling telling her that he was fighting a man over her.

Tracy ask if she was sleeping with her brother and got him in a mix up with her mess.

Candy was yelling no and crying on her knees to Tracy.

Tracy says no way, now she got to bury her brother. Her life is a mess Tracy wants to kill herself and give up.

Candy is crying and saying that she is sorry. She finally confesses to Tracy that she was cheating on her with her brother and he found out she gave him HIV.

Tracy ask why, because her brother was helping her get money.

You were getting greedy and didn't give a fuck Tracy says to Candy. She yells at her for her to leave and tell her time is going to catch up with her if she didn't change her life.

She tried to see if she would after what she went through with her coma for 2 months she had.

But she sees that Candy is all about herself and Candy is hard down saying please don't let her go she loves her.

Tracy says, "Bull shit you don't know how to love." She loved her for 6 years and she still don't see a change in her so she wants a divorce and to move on with her life. Tracy says it's time to move on and to get out.

Tracy gets a divorce and Candy was charged with murder and giving men and some woman HIV.

Candy is in prison for 25 years. Damn, that's sad. Like they say what goes around comes around.

She said Candy is going to get hers and that her time was gonna catch up with her.

Well as you see her time caught up with her and what the argument was about so not only is Tracy all alone again but she realized in life, you live and you learn.

She realizes that her life was going around in a circle that she had to turn around in her mind. She was crying asking, why did her life have to be this way. She was a good girl what was it that she had done to want to live the life of the streets. She was on her knees crying to God asking herself is it over I have full blown HIV. She saying to God she was telling people she had it.

She was looking back in her life as when she was a little girl and saying, God where did this little sweet girl go?

Some women in life don't realize what you do in front of your child, how it affects them as they get older. You would think that they don't remember what you do to them, well guess what? Kids do remember.

Tracy is seeing that now. All because she thought what her mom was doing when she was little, was cool. Things that were allowed around her, she saw and let it happen to herself.

Tracy is now remembering what a mess she had gotten into and that this is why things are happing to her. Her mother was wrong for doing things in front of her like that, knowing her daughter looked up to her as a role model.

I know her mother felt ashamed as she was getting herself clean, well tried to.

The mother died as well but before she passed away she did tell Tracy that she was sorry for all the things that had happened to her that she had allowed to happen.

You know how the saying goes, what you do on to others shall happen twice back on to you.

So she did get her friendship back with her mother but just for a little while, but by that time it was all too late for all of that. Tracy forgave her and grew up and had to move on with her life.

As you know, Tracy's book was a Bestseller and she made plenty of money off her books. She is still living her life as a Published Author.

Tracy also forgave Candy but they are not together. Candy had to be relocated to an area in the jail where HIV people were. Candy is still sleeping with other woman that have it in jail where she is.

Life is crazy, you make life as you experience it. You grow up and you learn even as an adult you still make more mistakes but Tracy wrote about people she new and things she went through.

Her story was written in hopes that people should not do things in front of a child that you don't want them to grow up doing; because they will pick up everything you are doing.

Tracy still have HIV, but is living with it with good medicine like the basketball player, Magic Johnson did.

You can see Tracy gave up on that fast life style. She's not rich and all, but she is happy in a nice Condo. You can say she maybe the next Mary Jane, something like the TV show that comes on.

Yes, she is into writing her books, and that's her lifestyle now and is mentoring young women that have low self-esteem. She is continuing her HIV counseling, one on one and group therapy.

She did get her life back together as a single woman. It seems like in order for things to get better in life, you have to stay away from the bad; and sometimes it's hard because you don't know who's good for you unless you can read that person. Only if God have given you a great gift that way people can't hurt you because you can already read their spirit.

So, to those that read this book I hope that it was good and that you look forward to reading more books from me this is the end thanks to all and good day, God Bless.

This Book was written in order for those to understand that you can catch anything if you don't use protection and that people you look up to aren't always a good role model.

This book is based on how you think you know a person but you really don't. This is a true story about a young lady that I knew, and a few people that I ran into in life that gave me a story to tell. Also things that I have seen as well as a lil girl

And no, none of these things happened to me. There was a time where things were rough and as I got older I saw people on Molly's and other drugs that this world has. Yes, people ask me but I was smart enough not to do what other people do. I did things on my own and yes I learned from it and yes I am living a better life.

The young woman is also living a better life well, she is a woman and a lot older than I am, but hey, as they say what goes around, comes around.